IT IS **IMPORTANT** TO BE HEALTHY.

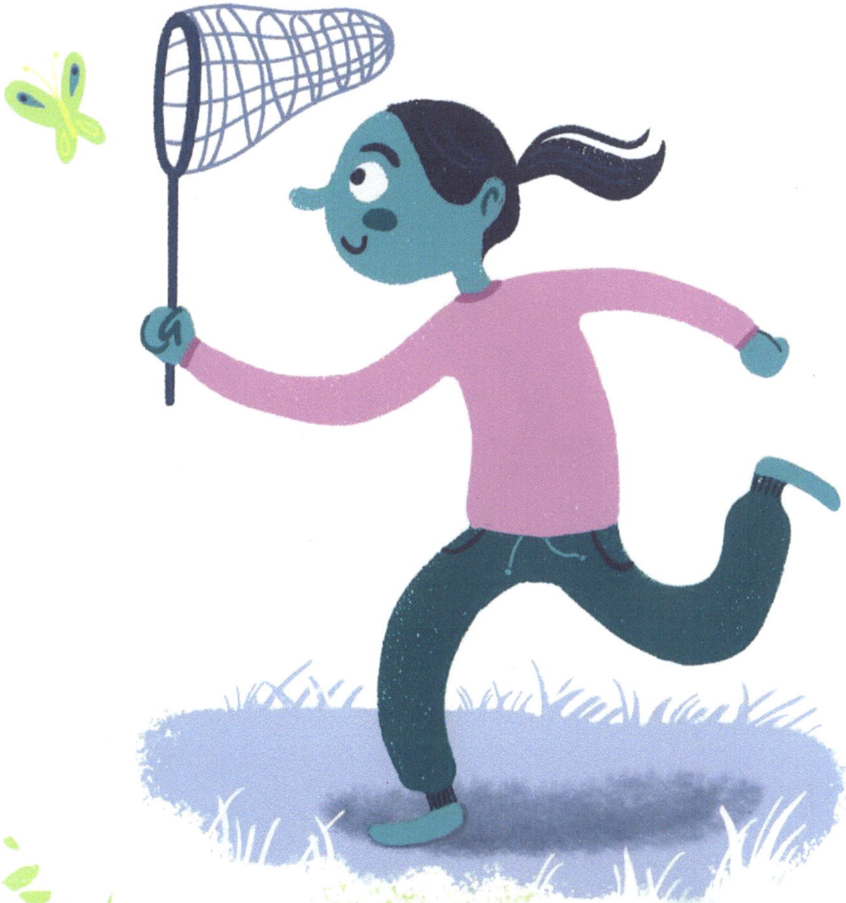

REGULAR MEDICAL EXAMS BY A DOCTOR

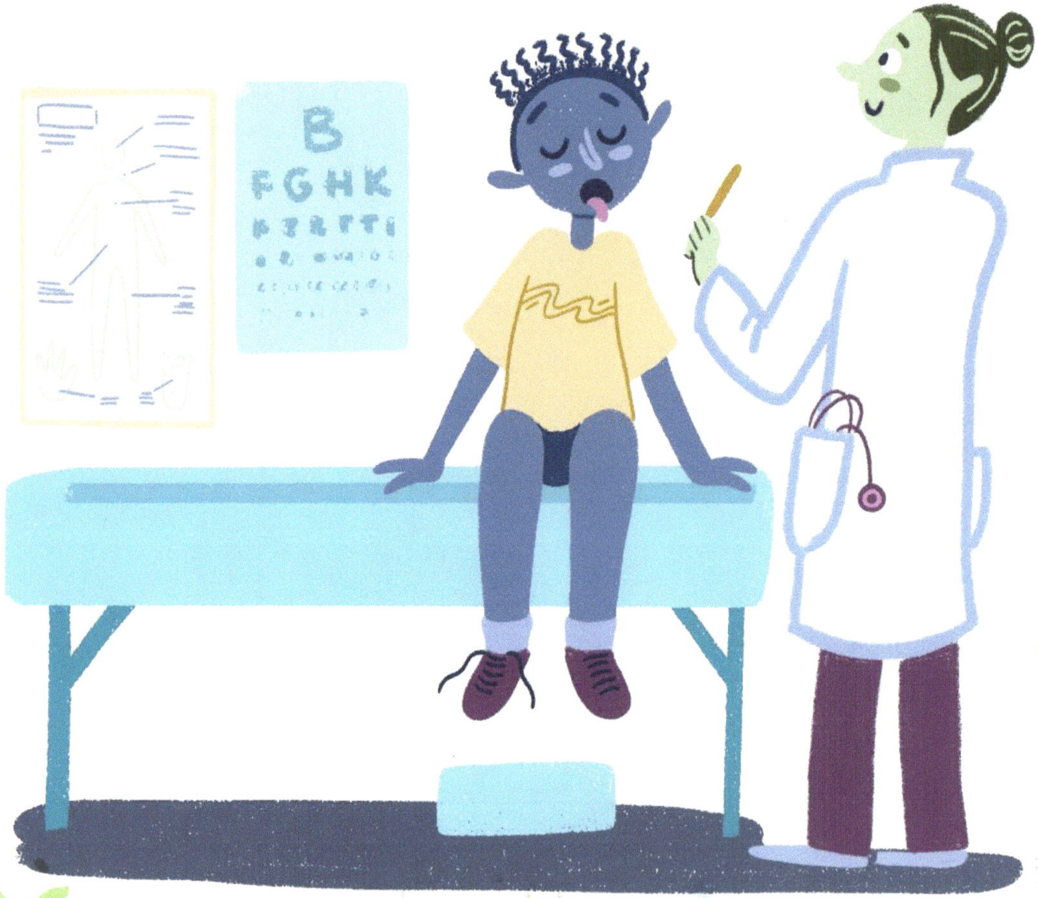

CHECK THE BODY FOR ANY SIGNS OF ILLNESS OR INJURY.

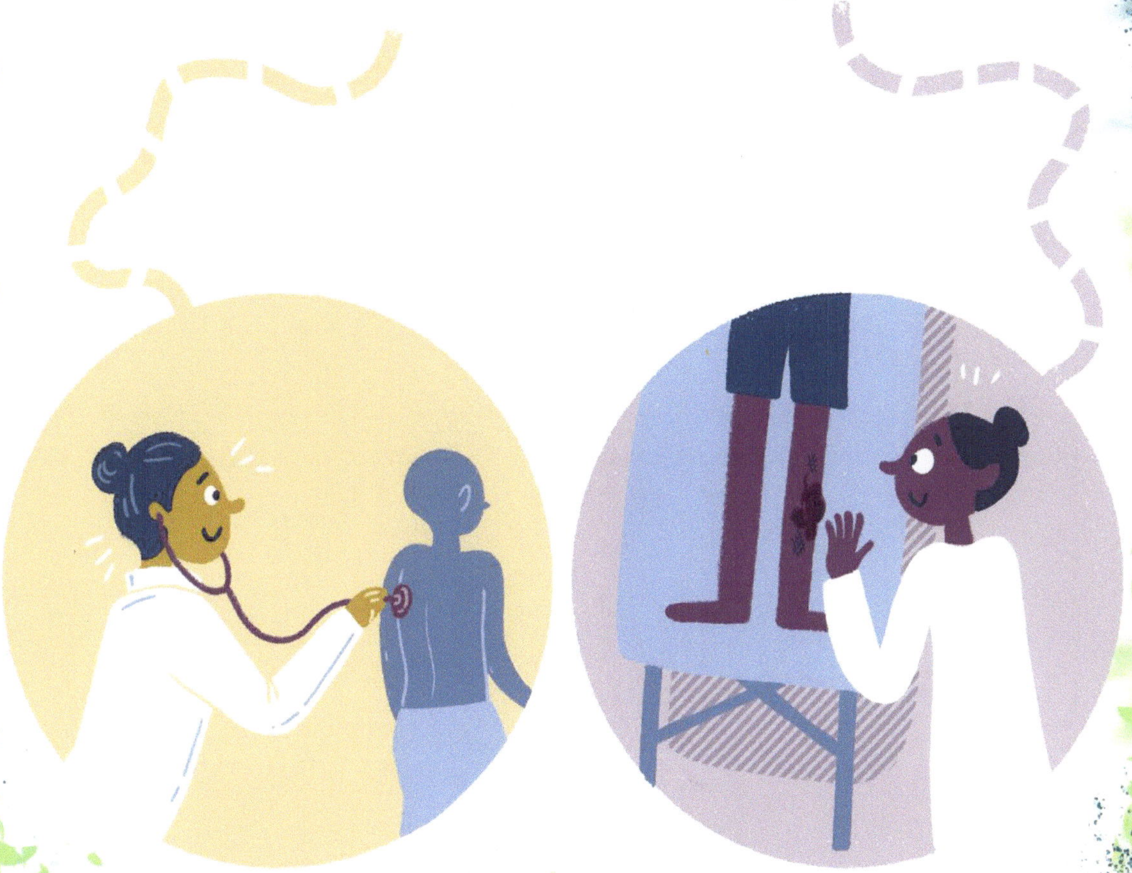

TESTS CAN BE PERFORMED TO PREVENT PROBLEMS.

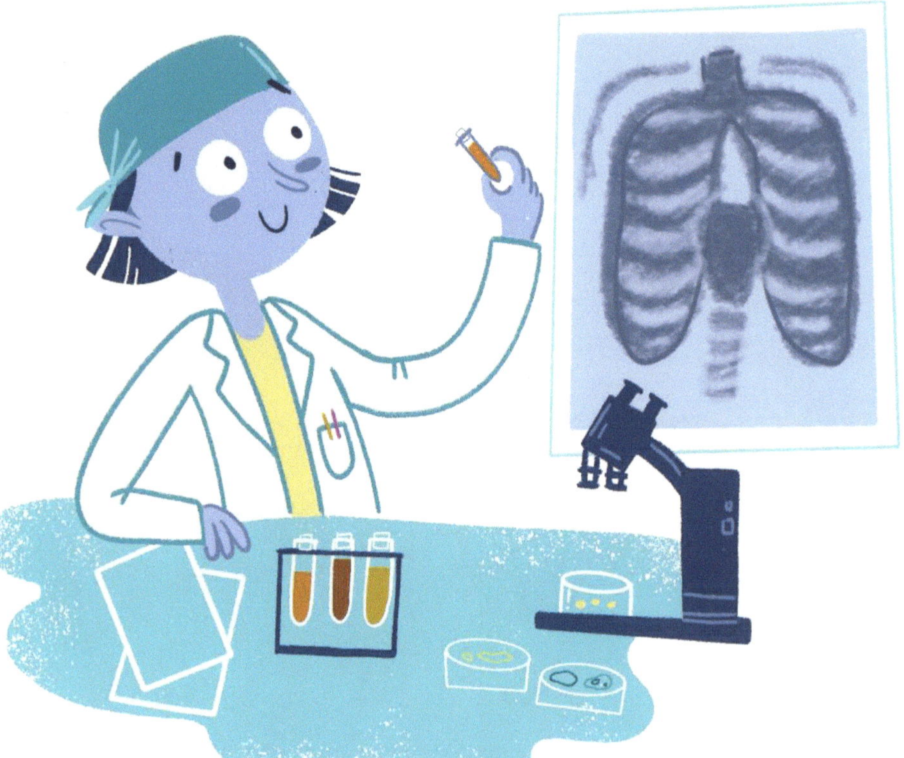

FOR EXAMPLE, TESTING THE HEART CAN DETECT POTENTIAL DISEASE.

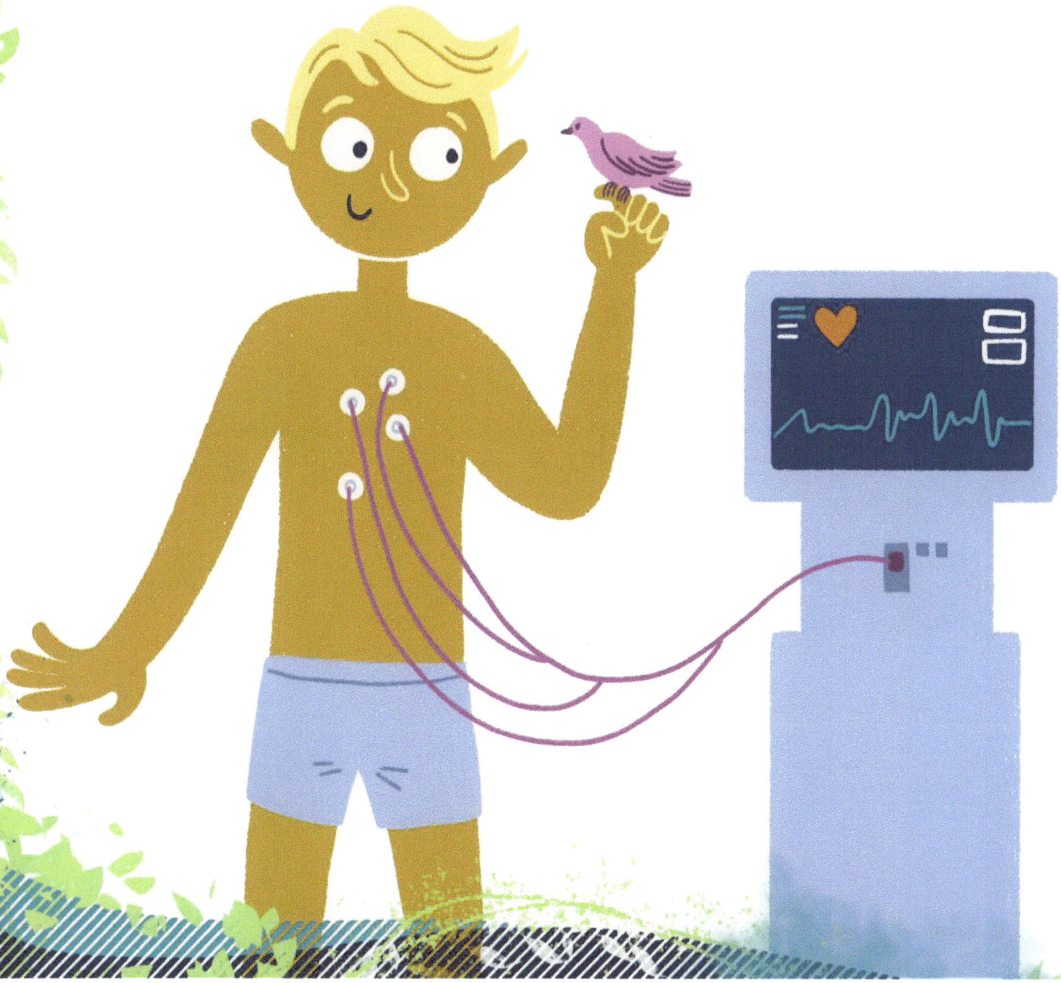

IF A **PROBLEM** IS
NOTICED **EARLY**,

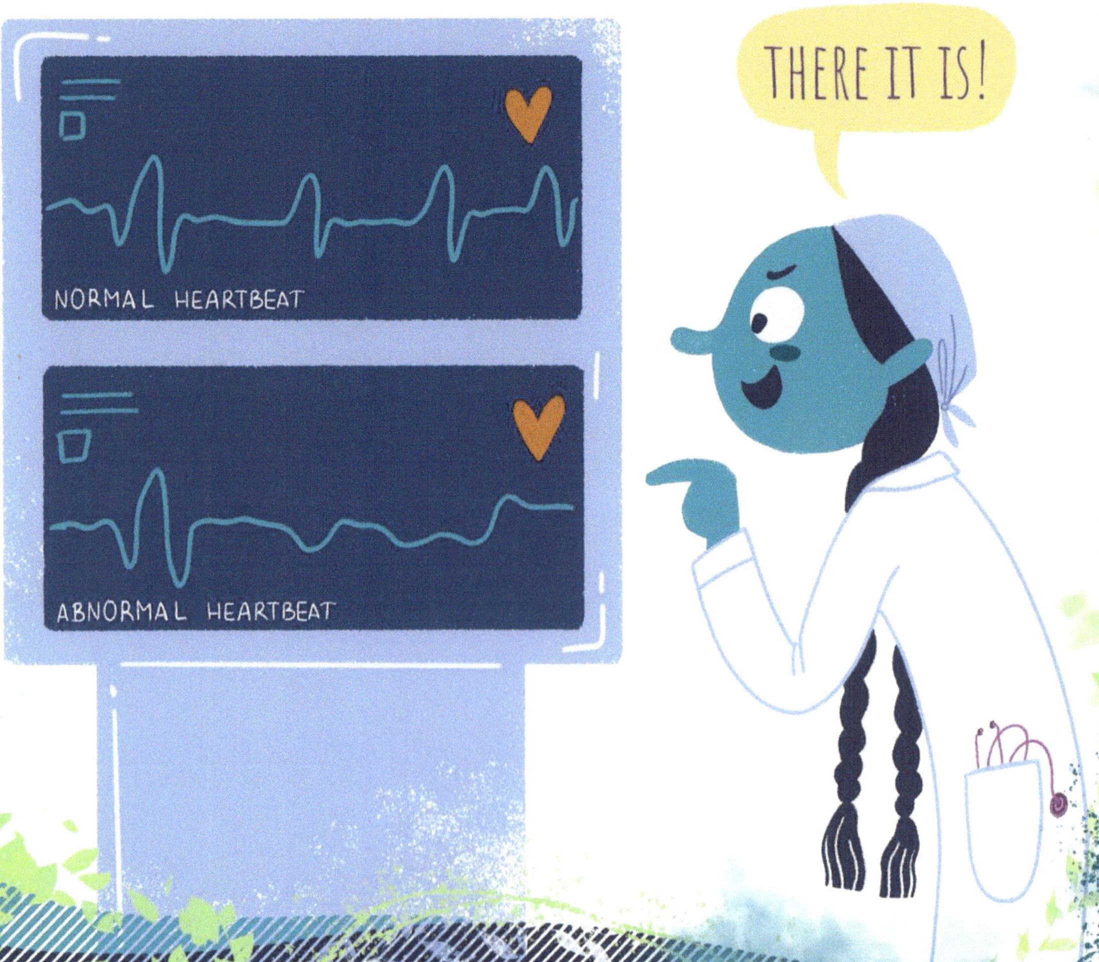

MEDICINE AND OTHER PRECAUTIONS CAN STOP IT FROM GETTING WORSE.

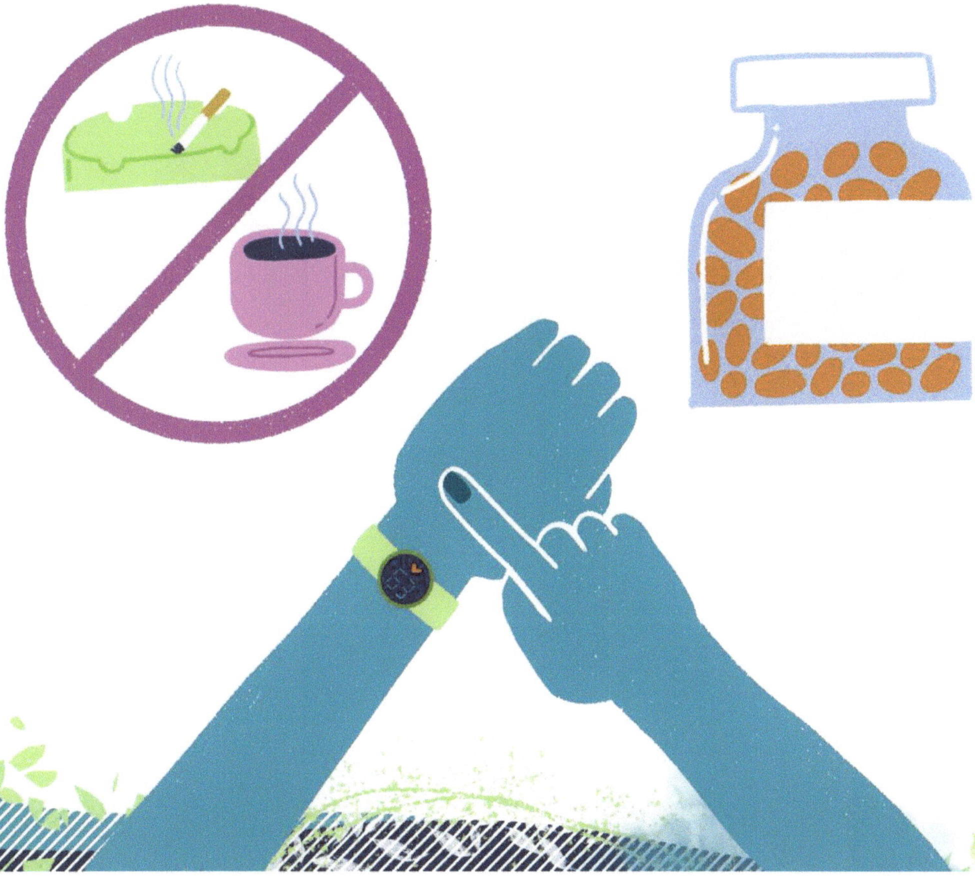

IF YOU DO GET SICK OR HURT

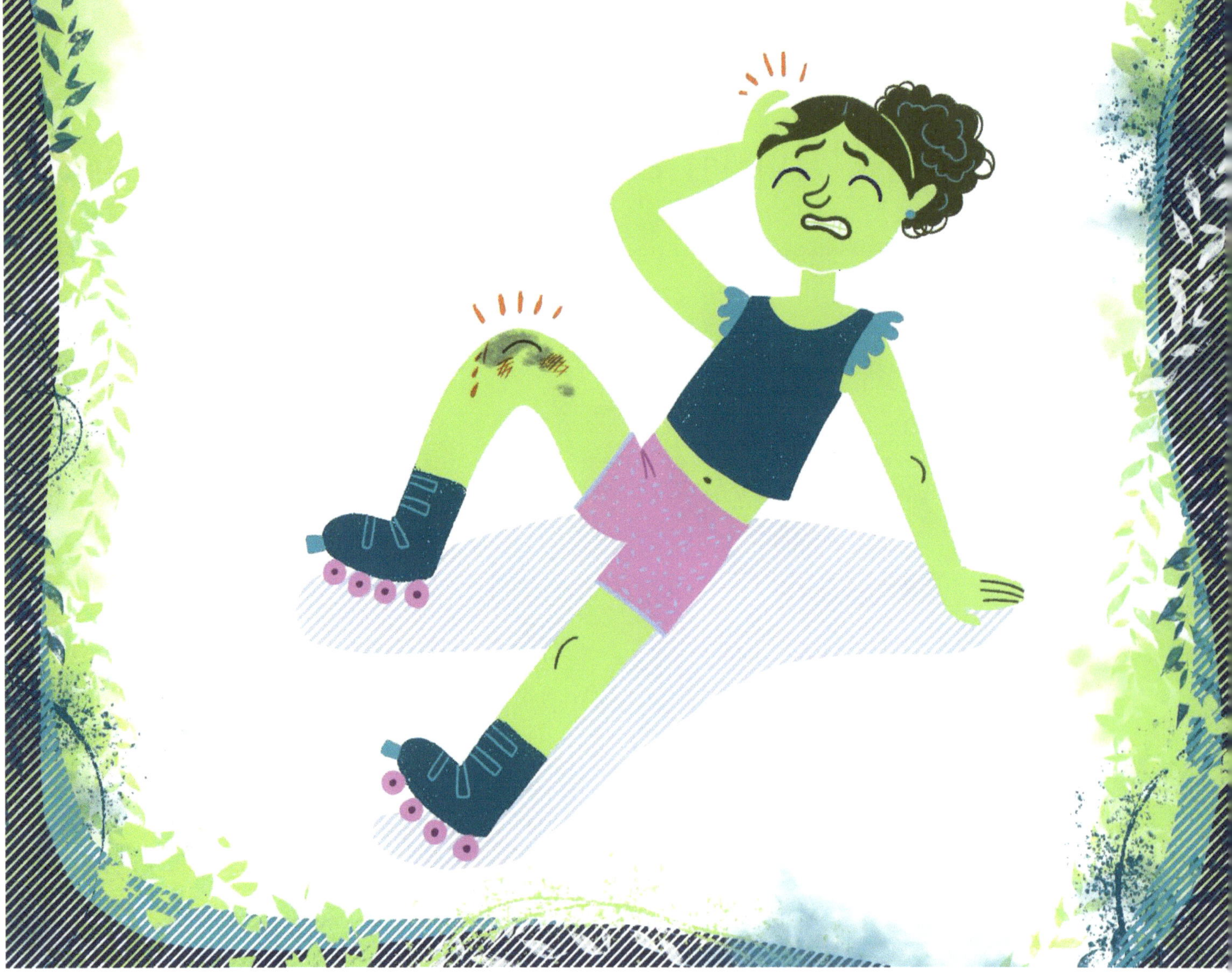

TESTS CAN HELP DETERMINE THE CAUSE.

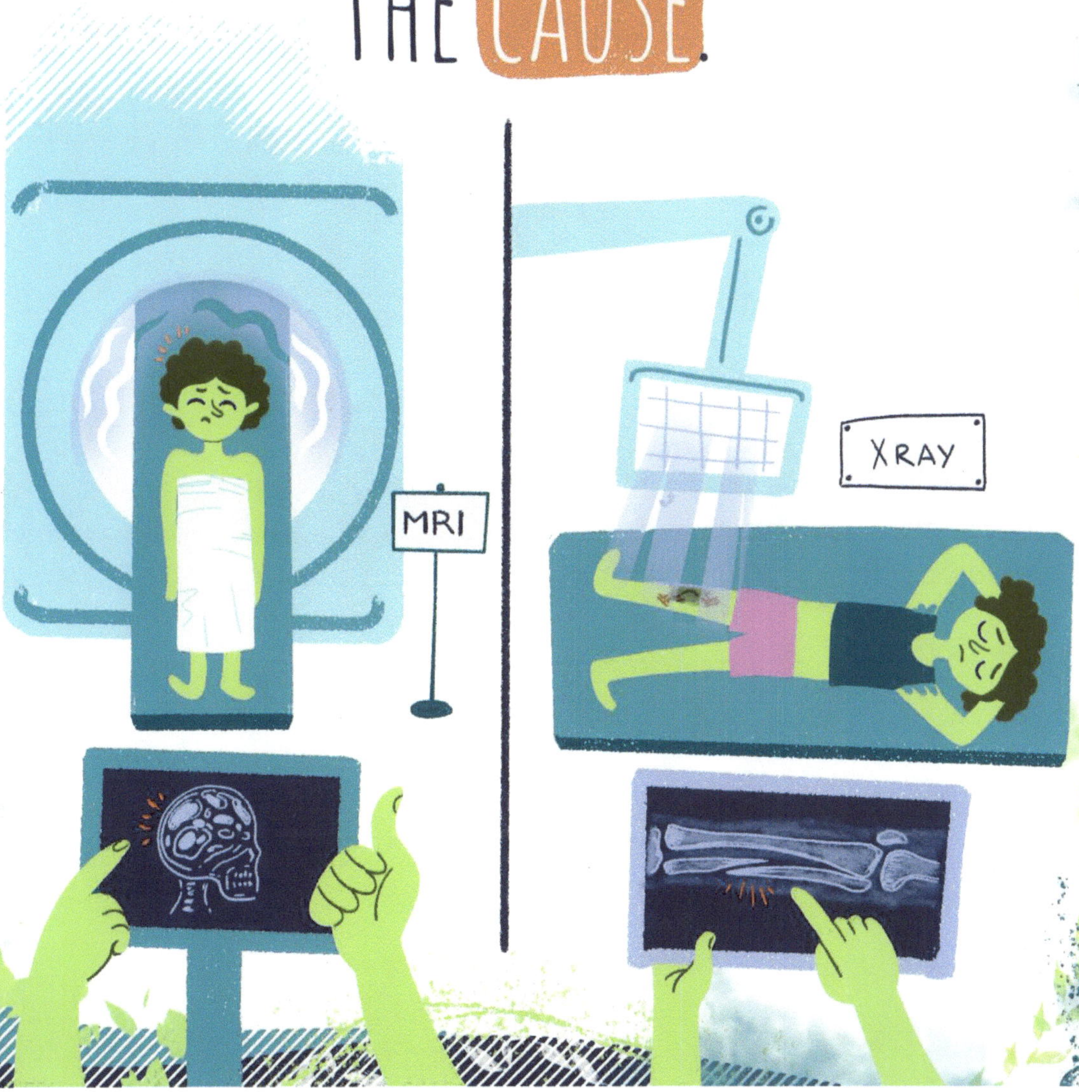

THESE TESTS ARE CALLED DIAGNOSTIC.

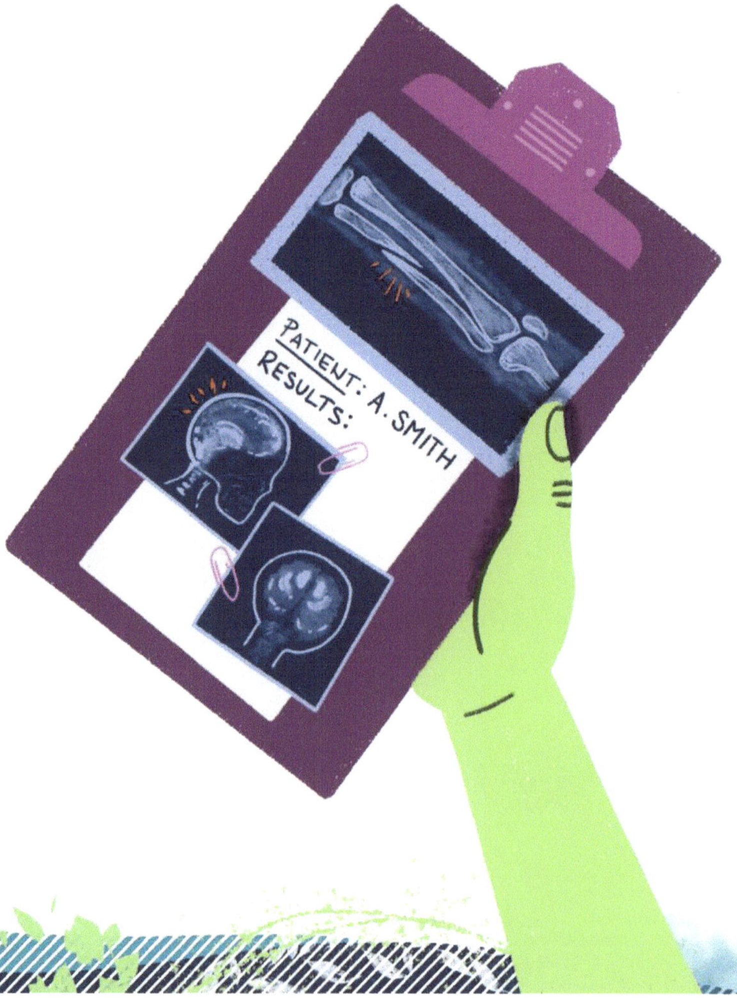

MANY OF THE TESTS WERE DEVELOPED BY BIOMEDICAL ENGINEERS.

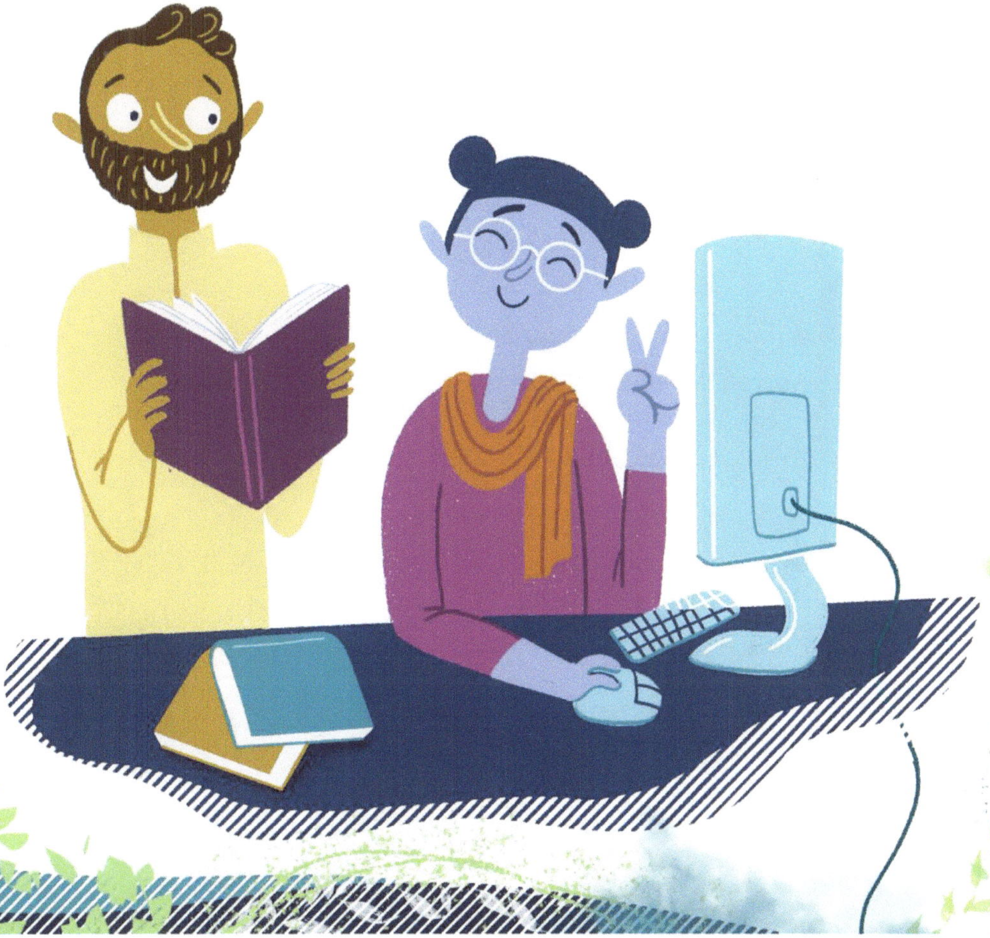

A BIOMEDICAL ENGINEER DESIGNS LAB TESTS,

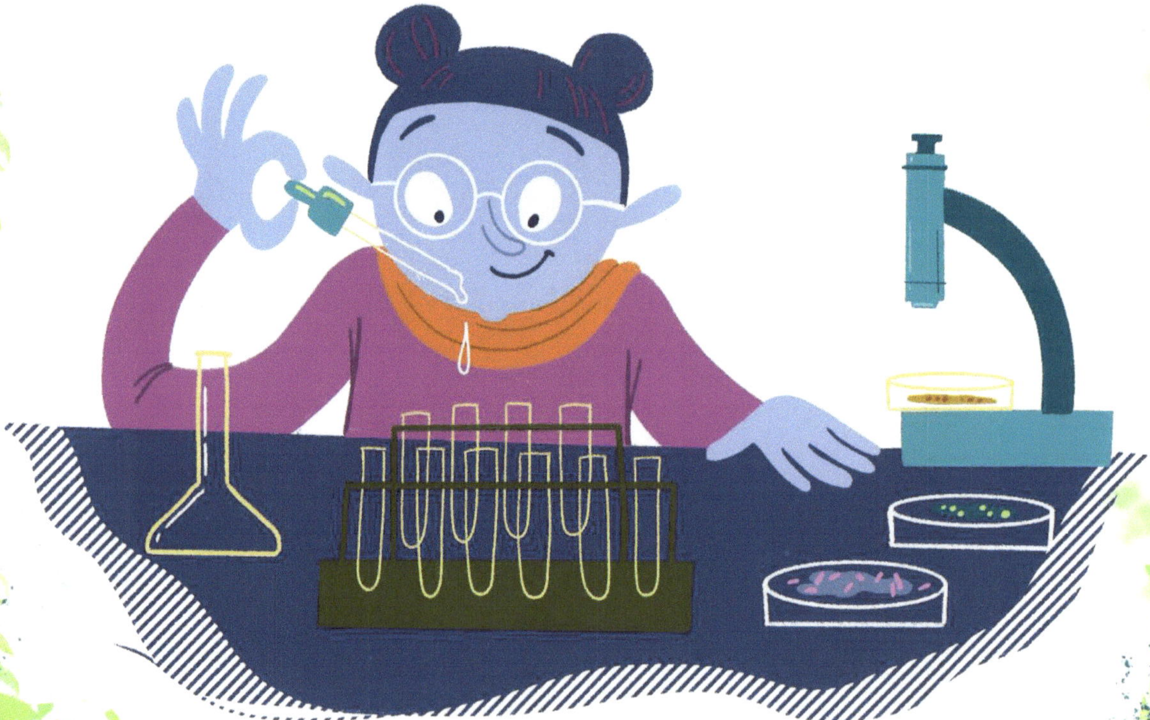

EQUIPMENT AND DEVICES.

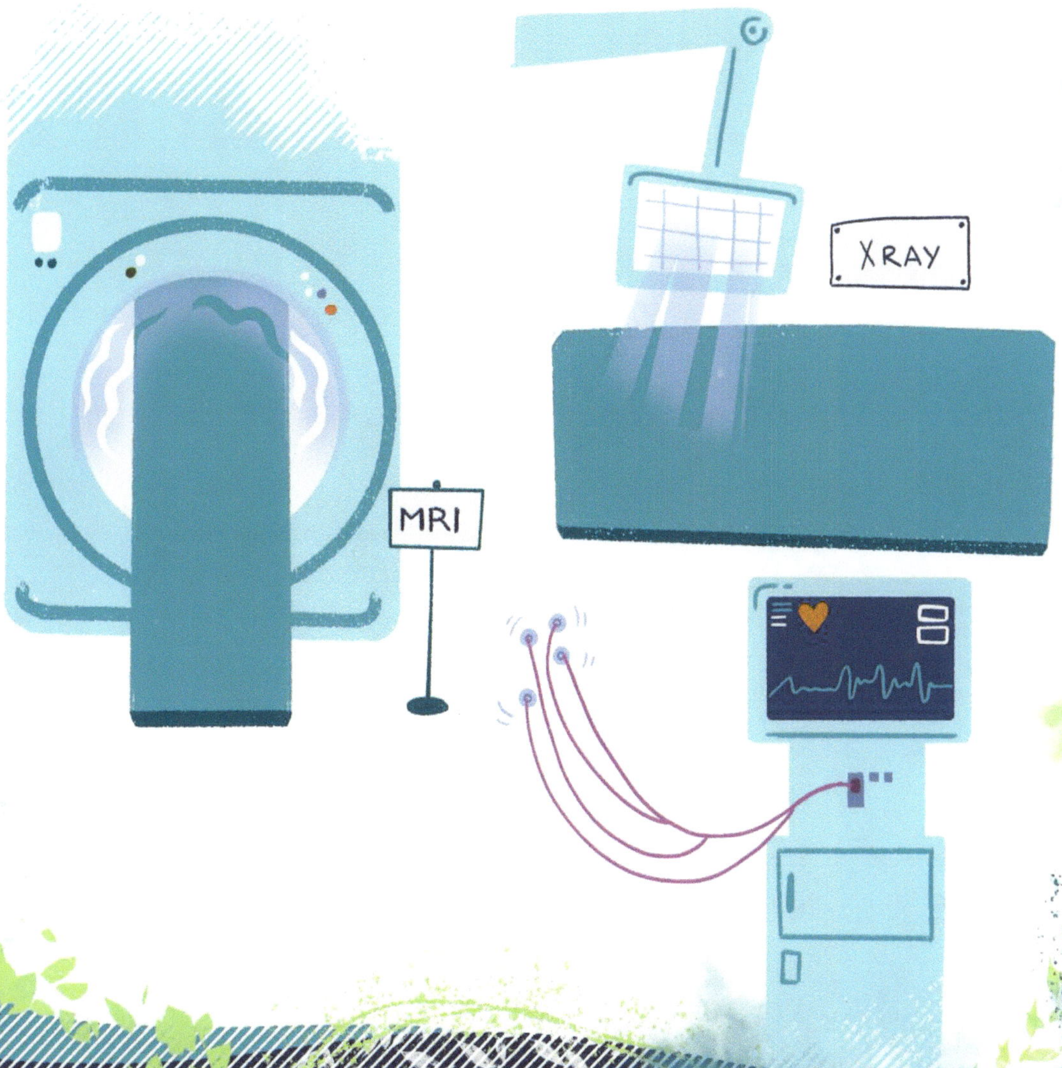

THEIR CREATIONS HELP DOCTORS

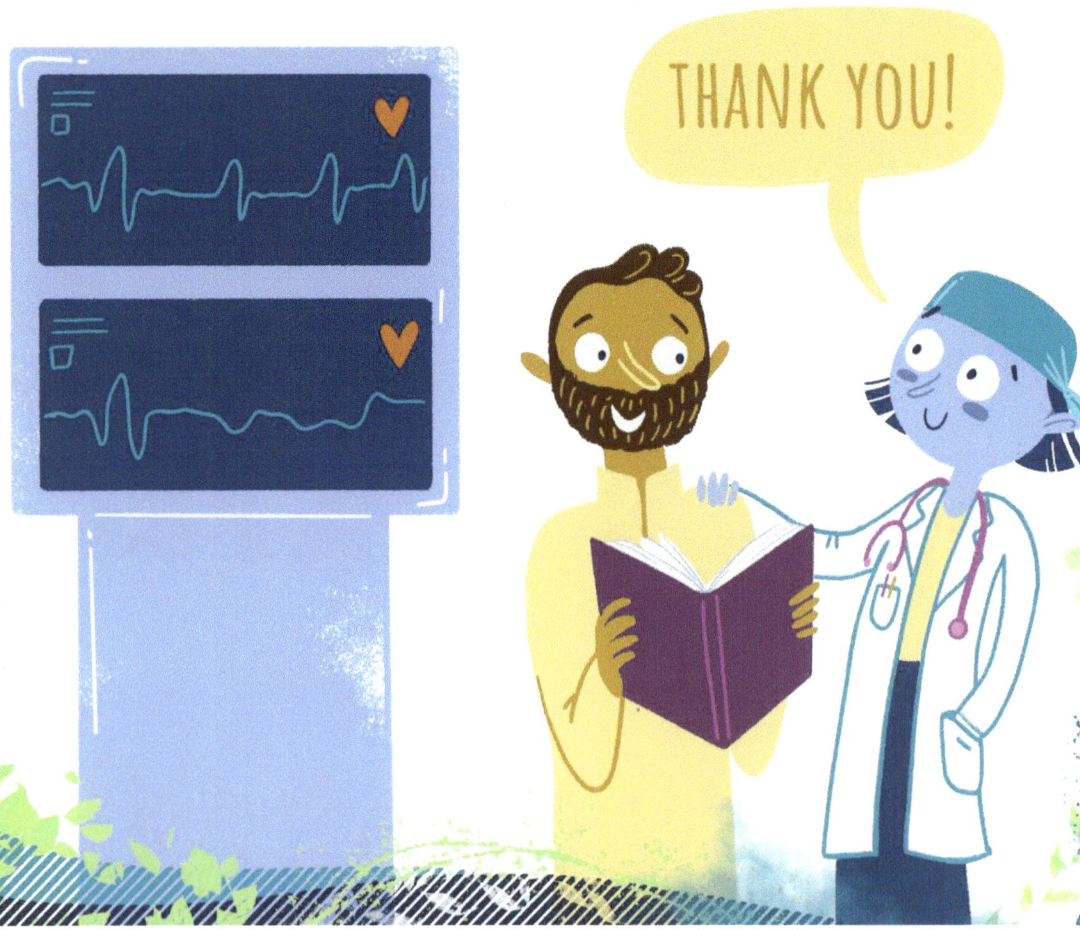

DECIDE WHAT IS BEST FOR YOUR HEALTH.

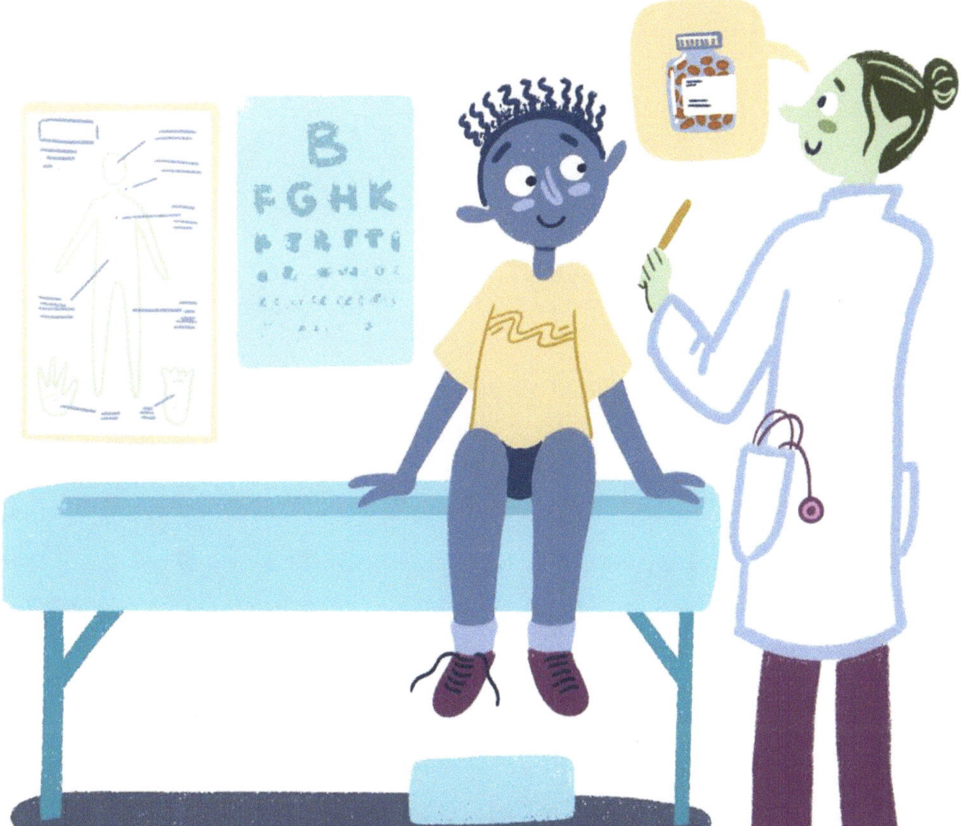

BIOMEDICAL ENGINEERS ALSO BUILD REPLACEMENT LIMBS,

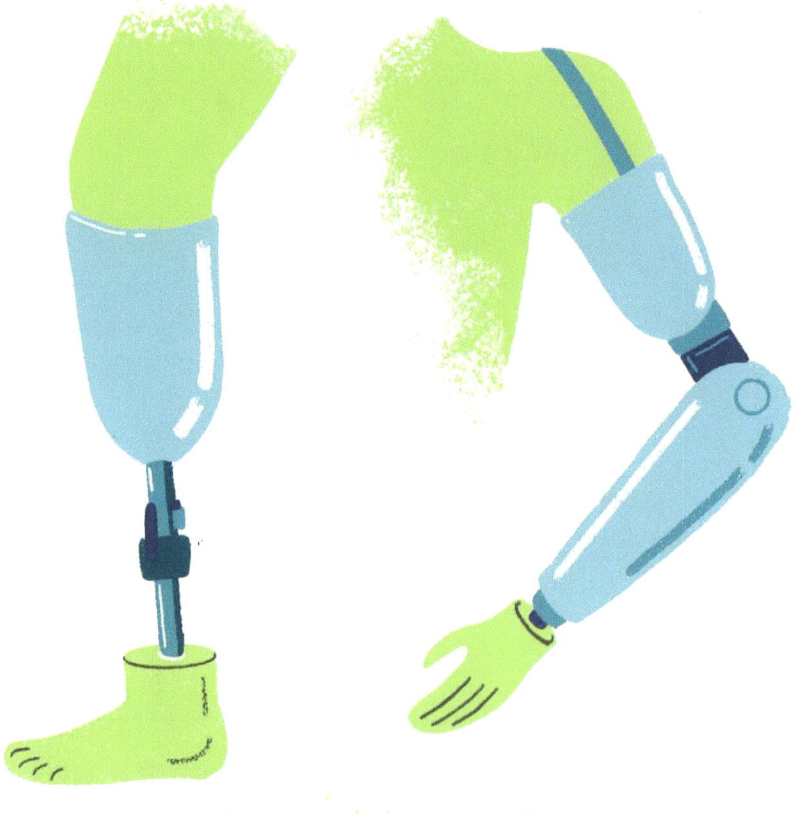

MAKE DEVICES TO CONTROL THE HEART

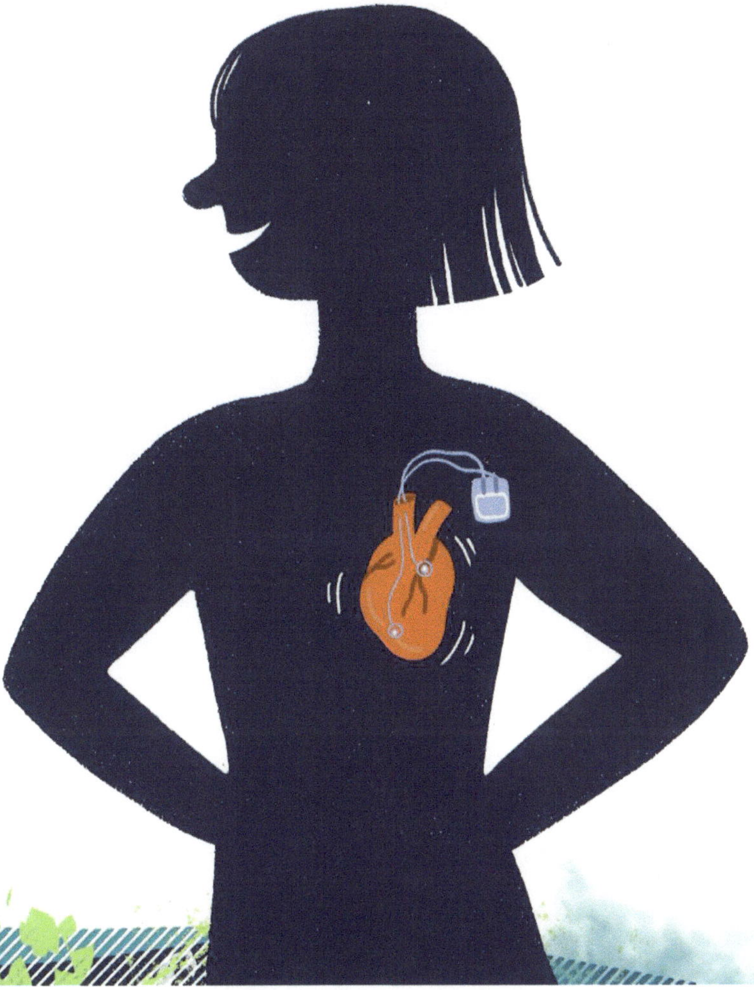

AND REGROW DAMAGED TISSUE.

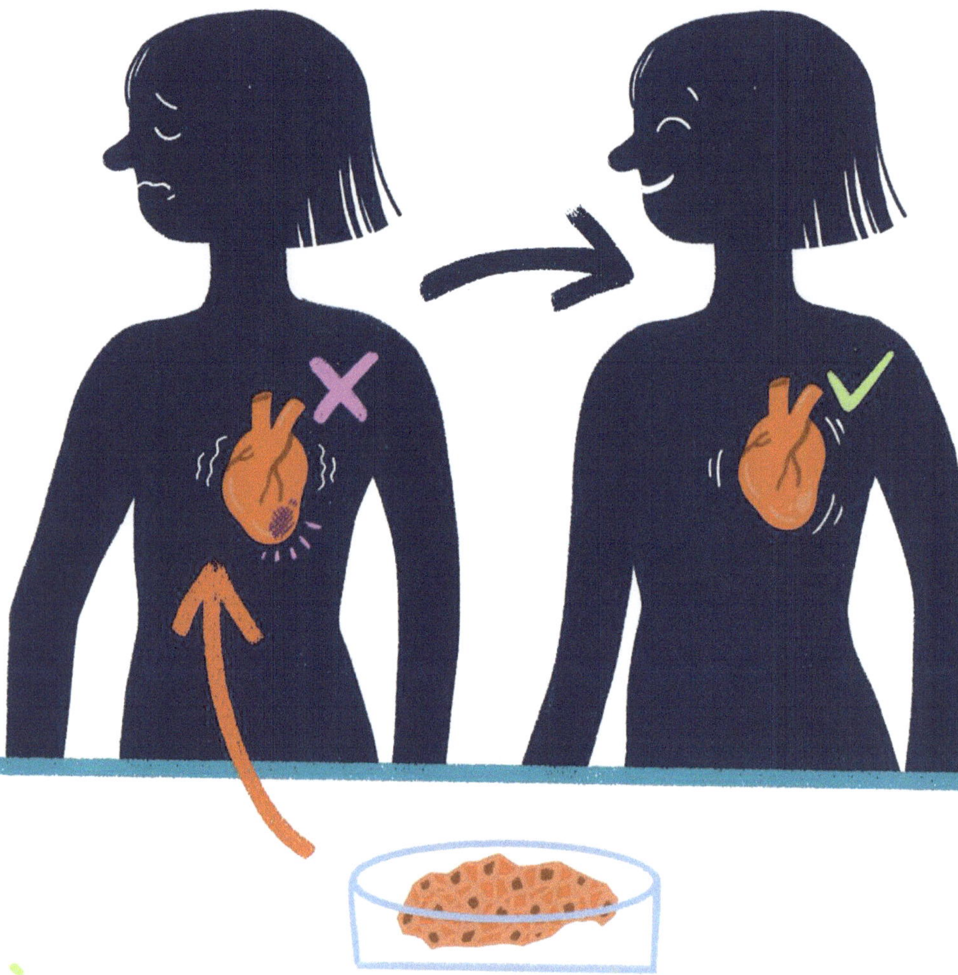

BIOMEDICAL ENGINEERING IS NECESSARY

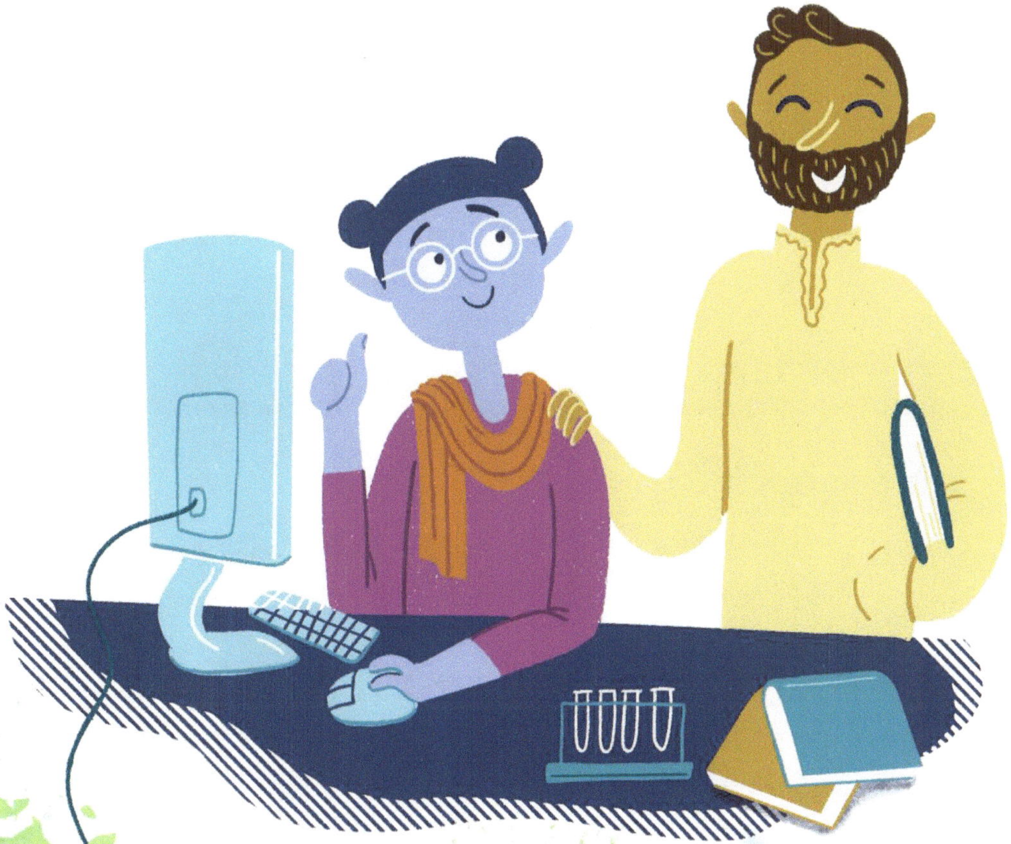

FOR IMPROVING HEALTHCARE.

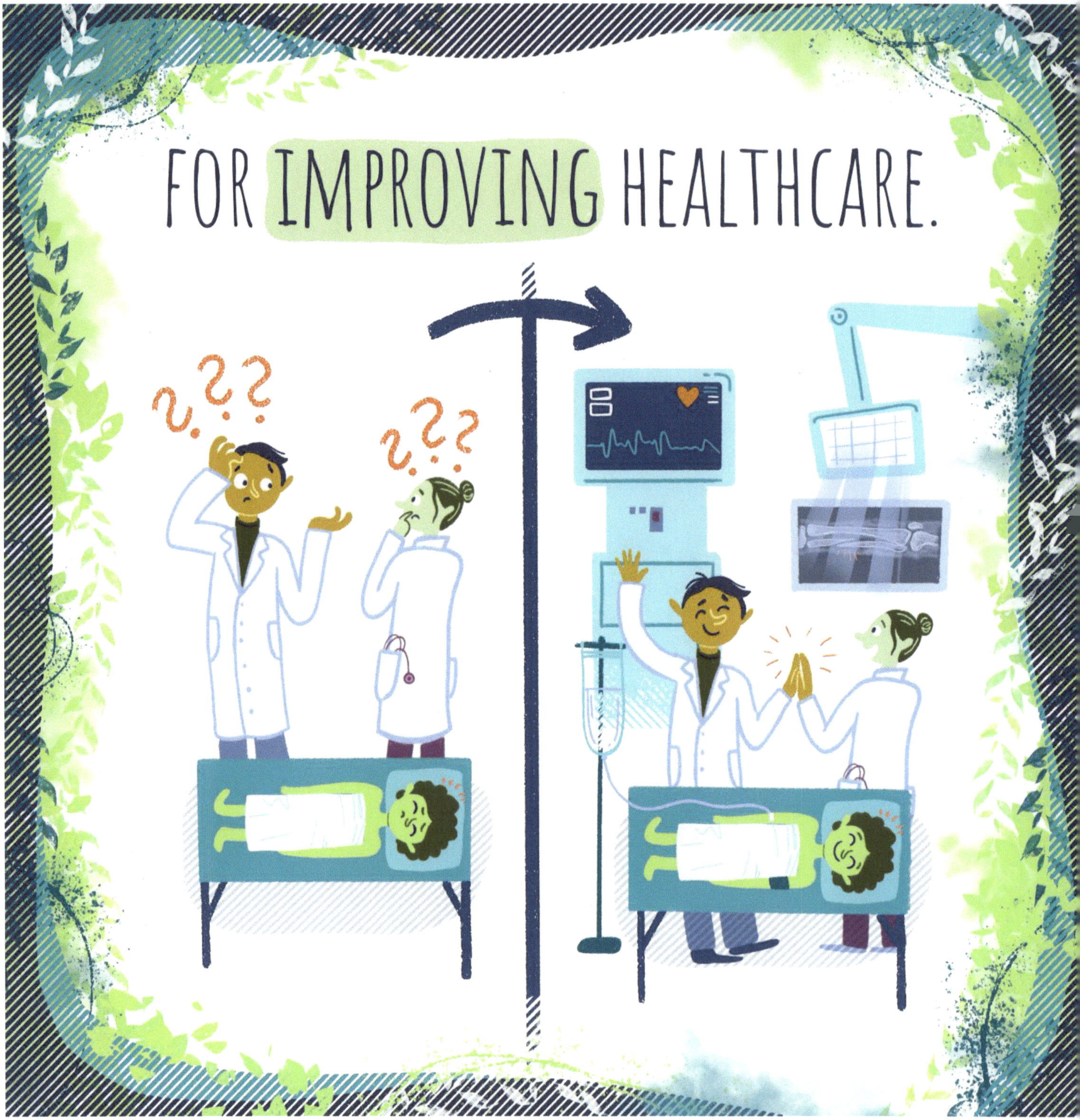

THEIR SCIENTIFIC DISCOVERIES

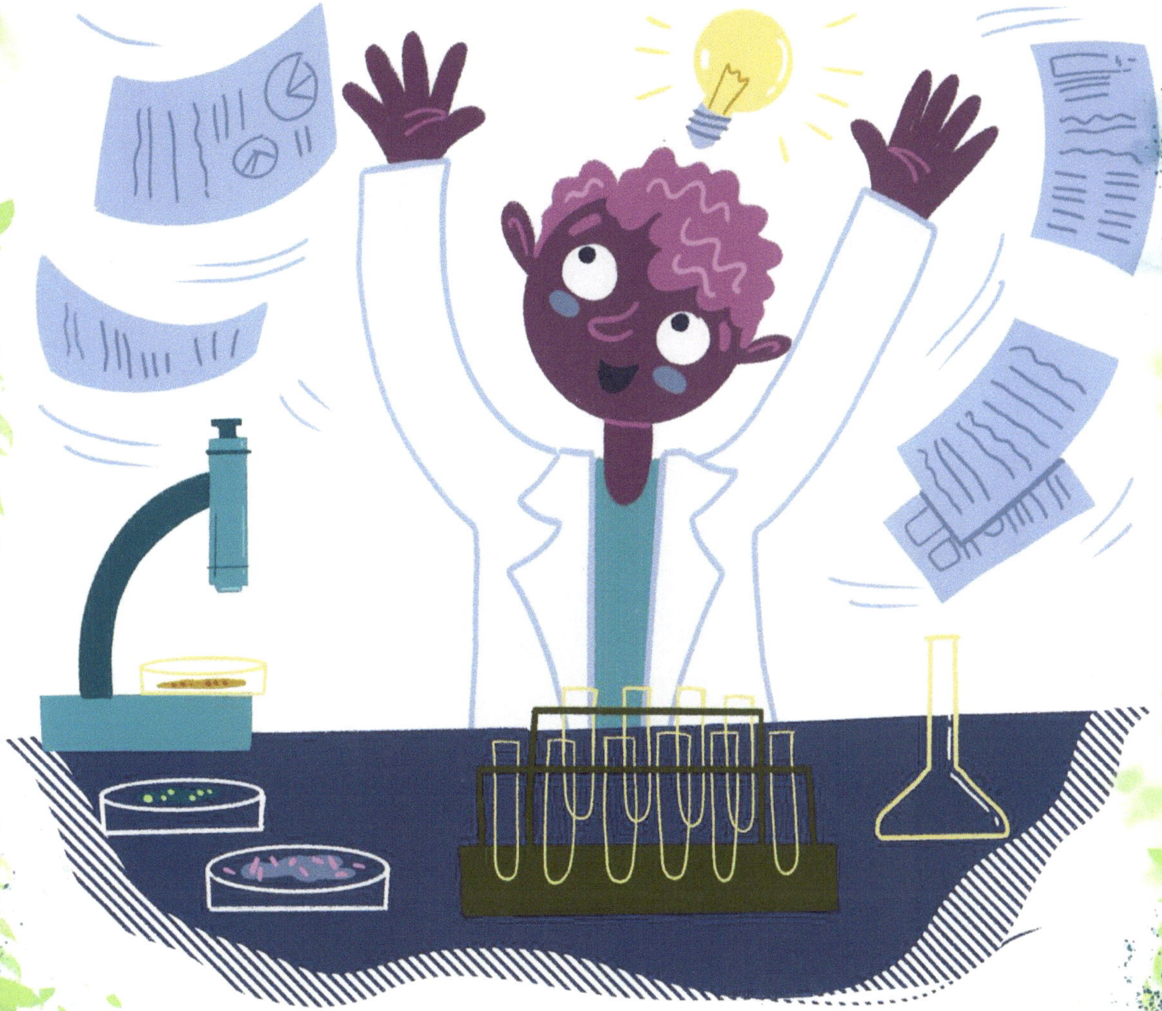

HELP US STAY HEALTHY FOR LONGER!

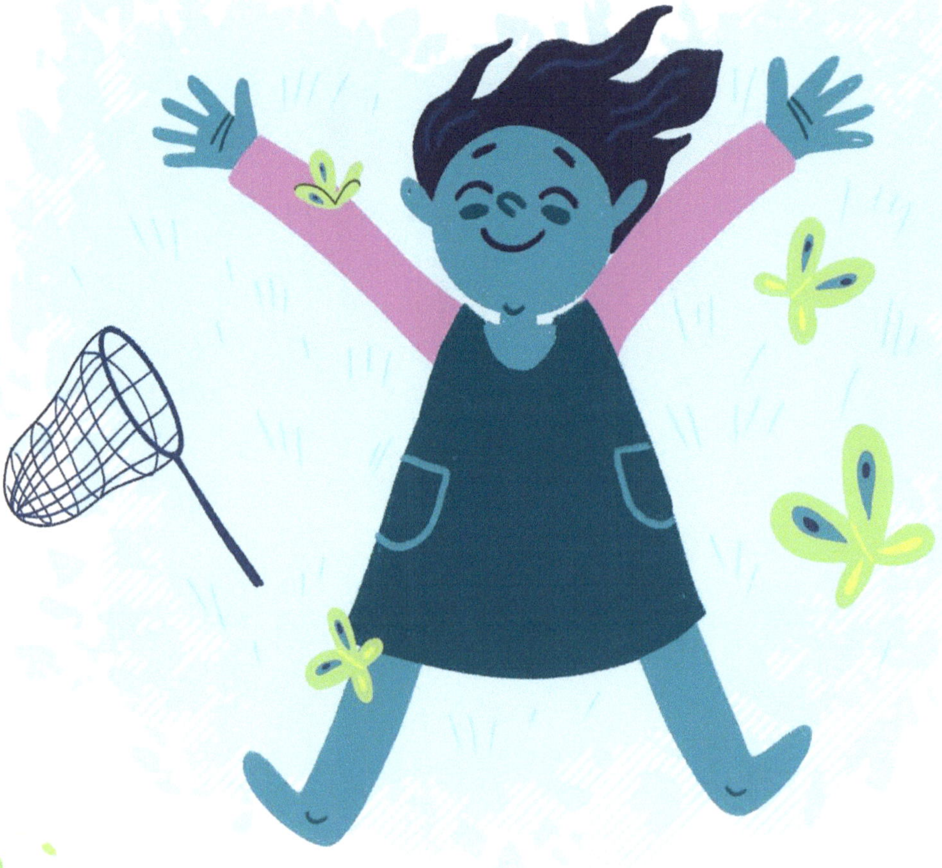

IT'S A GREAT **BIG** WORLD, WITH LOTS OF OPPORTUNITIES...

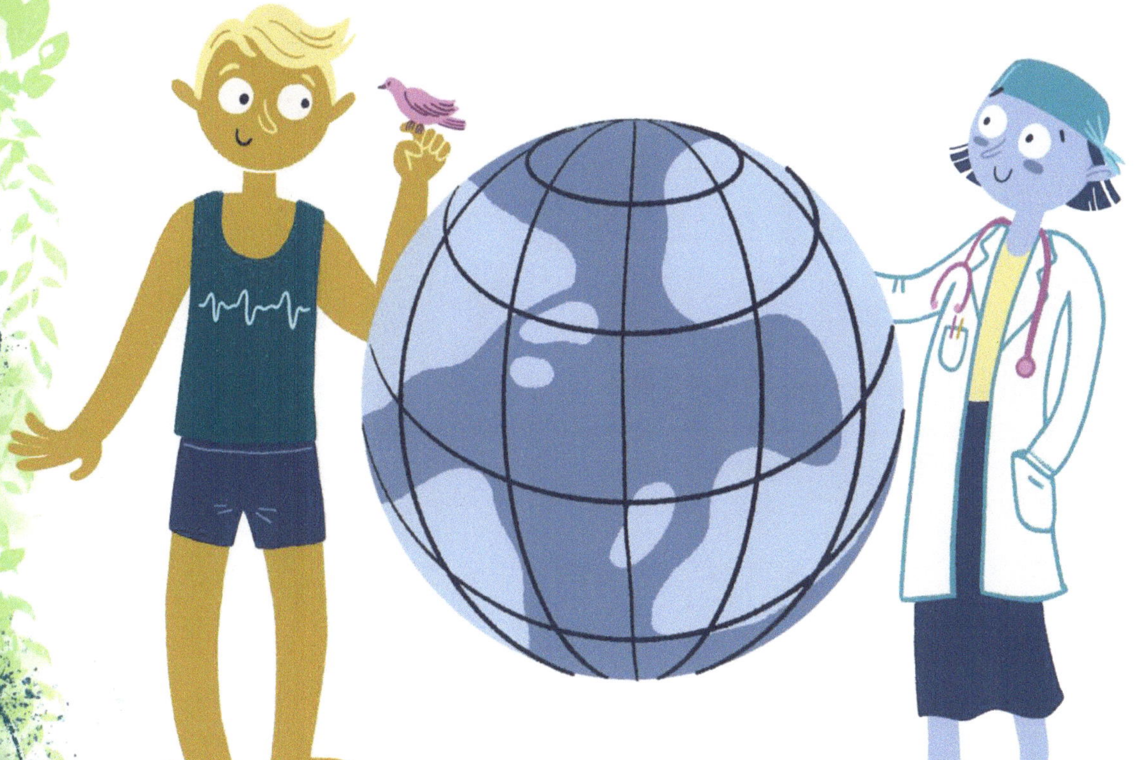

WHEN YOU GROW UP,
YOU CAN BE AN **ENGINEER!**

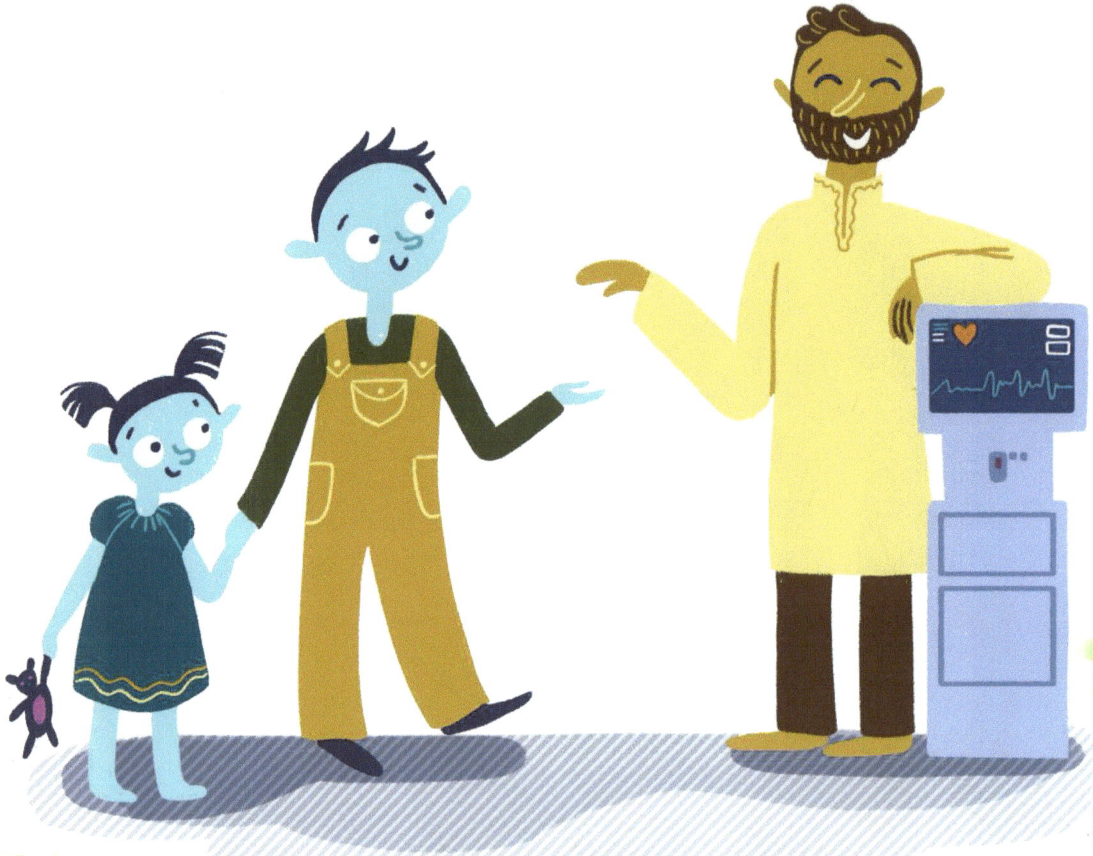

www.ingramcontent.com/pod-product-compliance
Lightning Source LLC
Chambersburg PA
CBHW051835210526
45473CB00005B/1881
9781721766871